Essential guide
for Beginners

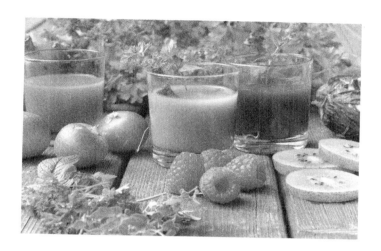

100+ juicing recipes for weight loss, detoxification, prevent aging and gaining energy

Glen Freeman

TABLE OF CONTENT

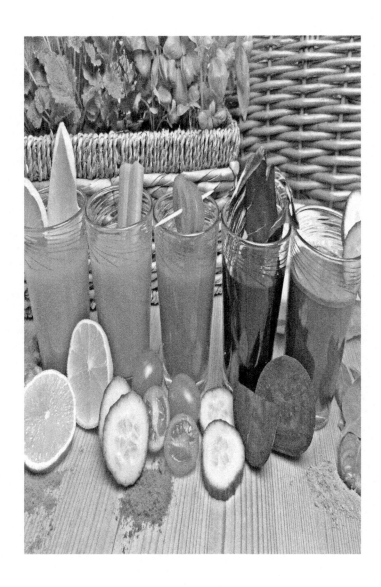

INTRODUCTION

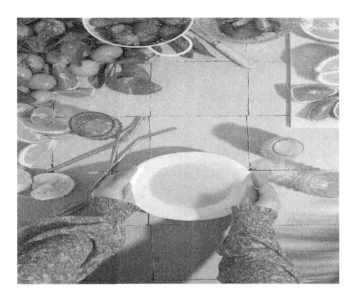

Welcome to the Essential Guide to Juicing Recipes for Beginners! Juicing has gained immense popularity in recent years as a powerful way to enhance health and well-being. Whether you're looking to shed some extra pounds, cleanse your body, slow down the aging process, or boost your energy levels, juicing can be an excellent addition to your wellness routine.

In this comprehensive guide, we have curated over 100 juicing recipes that are specifically designed to aid in weight loss, detoxification, preventing aging, and increasing energy levels. These recipes are not only delicious but also packed with essential nutrients, vitamins, and minerals that can nourish your body from within.

If you're new to juicing, don't worry! We will walk you through the basics, including how to choose the right ingredients, prepare your produce, and maximize the nutritional benefits of each recipe. You'll discover the importance of using fresh, organic ingredients and how to balance flavors to create a delightful juicing experience.

Whether you prefer fruity blends, green detoxifiers, or vibrant vegetable concoctions, this guide has something for everyone. We have carefully crafted recipes that combine a variety of fruits, vegetables, herbs, and spices to tantalize your taste buds while providing numerous health benefits.

So, grab your juicer, stock up on fresh produce, and get ready to embark on a journey of health, vitality, and flavor. Let's dive into the world of juicing and explore the endless possibilities of rejuvenating your body and nourishing your soul!

CHAPTER ONE

THE BASICS OF JUICING

Juicing has gained popularity in recent years as a convenient and efficient way to incorporate more fruits and vegetables into our diets. This process involves extracting the liquid or juice from fresh produce, leaving behind the fiber and pulp. By consuming freshly squeezed juice, we can enjoy a concentrated dose of essential vitamins, minerals, and antioxidants that can contribute to overall health and well-being. In this guide, we will explore the benefits of juicing and provide guidance on choosing the right juicer for your needs.

Understanding the Benefits of Juicing

1. Increased Nutrient Absorption: Juicing allows our bodies to quickly and easily absorb the nutrients from fruits and vegetables. Without the fiber, our digestive system can process the juice more efficiently, delivering a higher concentration of vitamins, minerals, and antioxidants directly into our bloodstream.

2. Enhanced Hydration: Juicing is an excellent way to stay hydrated since fruits and vegetables contain high water content. Additionally, the electrolytes

and minerals found in fresh juice can help replenish the body's fluids and maintain proper hydration levels.

3. Improved Digestion: The removal of fiber during the juicing process can benefit individuals with sensitive digestive systems. Consuming juice allows the body to absorb nutrients without the strain of breaking down and digesting fiber, making it easier on the digestive system.

4. Increased Energy Levels: The nutrient-rich nature of fresh juice can provide a natural energy boost. The vitamins, minerals, and enzymes present in juice support various bodily functions and help combat fatigue.

5. Detoxification and Cleansing: Juicing is often associated with detoxification and cleansing due to its potential to flush out toxins from the body. The high antioxidant content in fruits and vegetables can aid in neutralizing free radicals and supporting the body's natural detoxification processes.

How to Choose the Right Juicer for Your Needs

1. Consider the Type of Juicer: There are several types of juicers available on the market, each with its pros and cons. The main types include:

- Centrifugal Juicers: These juicers use high-speed spinning blades to extract juice from produce. They are generally more affordable but may produce heat and oxidation, potentially reducing the nutrient content of the juice.

- Masticating Juicers: Also known as cold-press juicers, masticating juicers crush and squeeze the juice from fruits and vegetables. They operate at lower speeds, minimizing heat and oxidation and preserving more nutrients. Masticating juicers are usually more expensive but offer higher juice quality.

- Citrus Juicers: Designed specifically for citrus fruits like oranges and lemons, these juicers are simple to use and clean. They are typically affordable and produce juice quickly.

- Twin Gear Juicers: These juicers use two interlocking gears to extract juice. They operate at low speeds and are known for producing high-quality juice with minimal oxidation. Twin gear juicers are generally more expensive and suitable for serious juicing enthusiasts.

2. Consider Ease of Use and Cleaning: Look for a juicer that is easy to assemble, disassemble, and clean. Juicers with fewer parts and dishwasher-safe components can save time and effort in the cleaning process.

3. Consider Noise Level: Some juicers can be quite noisy, especially centrifugal juicers with high-speed motors. If noise is a concern for you, consider masticating juicers or citrus juicers, which tend to operate more quietly.

4. Yield and Pulp Extraction: Different juicers vary in terms of juice yield and pulp extraction. Some juicers extract more juice from the same amount of produce, while others leave behind drier pulp. Consider the desired yield and consistency of the juice you prefer when choosing a juicer.

5. Additional Features: Some juicers come with extra features such as;

   multiple speed settings, reverse function, or attachments for making nut butter or sorbets. Assess your needs and preferences to determine if these features are essential for you.

6. Budget Considerations: Juicers can range in price from affordable to quite expensive. Set a budget that aligns with your requirements and expectations, considering the long-term benefits and frequency of juicing.

Remember to thoroughly research and read customer reviews before making a final decision. Consider your personal preferences, lifestyle, and the types of produce you plan to juice to choose the juicer that best fits your needs. With the right juicer, you can embark on a journey towards better nutrition and enjoy the many benefits of juicing.

Selecting Fresh and Organic Ingredients

When it comes to juicing, selecting fresh and organic ingredients is key to ensuring the highest quality and nutritional value of your juices. Here are some pointers to assist you in selecting the ideal ingredients:

1. Shop at local farmers' markets or organic stores: These are great places to find fresh, seasonal, and locally grown produce. Local farmers' markets often offer a wide variety of fruits and vegetables that are harvested at their peak ripeness, ensuring optimal flavor and nutrient content.

2. Look for organic certification: Organic produce is grown without the use of synthetic pesticides, herbicides, or genetically modified organisms (GMOs). Choosing organic ensures that your ingredients are free from harmful chemicals and are grown using sustainable farming practices.

3. Consider the season: Opt for fruits and vegetables that are in season. They tend to be fresher, tastier, and more nutritious compared to

out-of-season produce. Seasonal produce is also more likely to be locally sourced, reducing the carbon footprint associated with transportation.

4. Inspect the quality: Examine the appearance and texture of the ingredients. Choose fruits and vegetables that are firm, vibrant in color, and free from blemishes, bruises, or signs of decay. Fresh herbs should have a strong aroma, indicating their freshness.

5. Go for ripe produce: Ripe fruits and vegetables not only taste better but also contain higher levels of nutrients. For instance, fully ripened fruits have higher antioxidant levels. However, be mindful that overripe produce may not store well, so plan your juicing accordingly.

Preparing and Cleaning Your Produce

Properly preparing and cleaning your produce is essential to remove any dirt, bacteria, or pesticides that may be present. Follow these steps to ensure your ingredients are safe to consume:

1. Wash your hands: Before handling any produce, wash your hands thoroughly with soap and water to minimize the risk of cross-contamination.

2. Rinse with water: Rinse your fruits and vegetables under cool running water to remove any surface dirt, pesticides, or residues. Use a

vegetable brush to gently scrub the skins of produce with firm surfaces, such as cucumbers or apples.

3. Use a natural produce wash: Consider using a natural produce wash or a mixture of water and vinegar to further reduce bacteria and remove wax or pesticide residues. Follow the instructions on the produce wash bottle or soak the produce in the solution for a few minutes before rinsing again.

4. Dry before juicing: After rinsing, pat dry or air-dry your ingredients using a clean cloth or paper towels. Moisture can dilute the flavor of your juices and contribute to faster spoilage.

Maximizing the Nutritional Value of Your Juices

To get the most out of your juices and retain their nutritional value, keep the following factors in mind:

1. Juice immediately: Freshly made juices are rich in vitamins, minerals, and enzymes. To maximize their nutritional content, consume your juices immediately after preparation. Oxidation and nutritional loss may result from exposure to air and light.

2. Store properly: If you need to store your juices, do so in airtight glass containers in the refrigerator.

Oxygen and light can degrade the nutritional value, so minimize exposure by filling the container to the brim and using dark-colored glass bottles or containers.

3. Drink on an empty stomach: Consuming juices on an empty stomach allows for better absorption of nutrients. Wait for at least 30 minutes before having a meal after drinking your juice.

4. Experiment with variety: Include a diverse range of fruits and vegetables in your juices to benefit from a wide array of nutrients. Different fruits and vegetables offer different vitamins, minerals, antioxidants, and phytochemicals, so mixing them up can maximize the nutritional diversity of your juices.

5. Consider adding superfoods: Boost the nutritional value of your juices by incorporating nutrient-dense superfoods like spinach, kale, ginger, turmeric, chia seeds, or wheatgrass. These ingredients provide an extra dose of vitamins, minerals, and antioxidants.

Remember, juicing can be a great way to increase your intake of fruits and vegetables, but it should not replace whole foods in your diet. It is important to maintain a balanced diet that includes a variety of foods from all food groups to ensure you receive a wide range of nutrients.

Juicing for weight loss has gained significant popularity in recent years as a potential strategy to support healthy weight management. Juicing involves extracting the juice from fresh fruits and vegetables, which provides a concentrated dose of nutrients while removing the insoluble fiber. Proponents of juicing believe that this process can help increase nutrient intake, promote detoxification, and support weight loss efforts. However, it's important to approach juicing as part of a balanced diet and lifestyle, rather than relying on it as a sole weight loss solution.

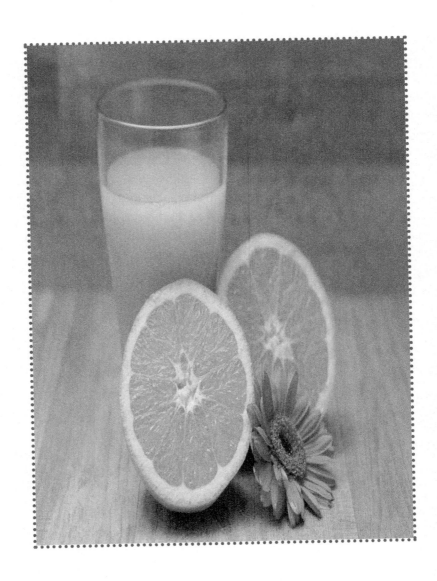

CHAPTER TWO

The Role of Juicing in Weight Management

1. Increased Nutrient Intake: Juicing allows you to consume a variety of fruits and vegetables in a convenient and easily digestible form. These nutrient-rich juices provide vitamins, minerals, antioxidants, and phytonutrients, which are essential for overall health and well-being. By incorporating a wide range of fruits and vegetables in your juices, you can enhance your nutrient intake and support your body's natural functions.

2. Reduced Caloric Intake: Juicing can help reduce overall caloric intake, as it often replaces higher-calorie beverages like soda or processed juices. Additionally, juicing can be used as a meal replacement or as a way to incorporate more low-calorie, nutrient-dense foods into your diet. By replacing a high-calorie meal with a balanced, nutrient-rich juice, you may create a calorie deficit, which can contribute to weight loss.

3. Hydration: Proper hydration is essential for weight management. Juicing can be an effective way to increase your fluid intake, as fruits and vegetables have high water content. Staying hydrated helps regulate appetite, supports

digestion, and aids in the elimination of toxins, all of which can positively impact weight management efforts.

4. Detoxification: Juicing is often associated with detoxification or cleansing. While the body has its built-in detoxification system through the liver and kidneys, incorporating fresh juices into your diet can support these natural processes. Juices rich in antioxidants, such as those containing dark leafy greens, citrus fruits, and berries, can help neutralize harmful free radicals and support the elimination of toxins from the body.

Key Ingredients for Weight Loss Juices

1. Leafy Greens: Dark leafy greens like spinach, kale, and Swiss chard are excellent additions to weight loss juices. They are low in calories and high in nutrients, including vitamins A, C, and K, as well as folate, iron, and fiber. Leafy greens can help boost metabolism, promote satiety, and provide essential nutrients for overall health.

2. Citrus Fruits: Citrus fruits like oranges, grapefruits, and lemons are rich in vitamin C and antioxidants. They add a refreshing flavor to juices while providing a natural sweetness. Citrus fruits also contain soluble fiber, which can help regulate

blood sugar levels and support weight management.

3. Berries: Berries such as strawberries, blueberries, and raspberries are packed with antioxidants, vitamins, and minerals. They are low in calories and high in fiber, making them ideal for weight loss juices. Berries also provide natural sweetness and can help satisfy cravings for sweets.

4. Cucumber: Cucumbers are hydrating and low in calories, making them an excellent ingredient for weight loss juices. They add a refreshing taste and contribute to the overall volume of the juice without significantly increasing the calorie content. Cucumbers also contain silica, which is beneficial for skin health.

5. Celery: Celery is a low-calorie vegetable that adds a unique flavor to juices. It is rich in water content, fiber, and vitamins, particularly vitamin K and potassium. Including celery in your weight loss juices can provide a refreshing and hydrating element to your beverage.

6. Ginger: Ginger has been used for centuries for its medicinal properties and is commonly added to juices for its flavor and potential health benefits. It has anti-inflammatory properties and may help

improve digestion and metabolism, which can indirectly support weight loss efforts.

35 delicious recipes for weight loss

Here's a comprehensive guide to the ingredients and procedures for delicious recipes that can support your weight loss goals:

1. **Green Detox Blast**:

Ingredients:
- 1 cucumber
- 2 cups spinach
- 1 green apple
- 1 lemon
- 1-inch ginger

Procedure:
a. Wash all the ingredients thoroughly.
b. Peel the cucumber and ginger, and remove the core from the green apple.
c. Cut the cucumber, green apple, and lemon into chunks.
d. Place all the ingredients in a juicer and extract the juice.
e. Stir the juice well and serve chilled.

2. **Berry Blast**:

Ingredients:
- 1 cup strawberries

- 1 cup blueberries
- 1 cup raspberries
- 1 cup almond milk
- 1 tablespoon chia seeds

Procedure:
a. Rinse all the berries under running water.
b. In a blender, combine the strawberries, blueberries, raspberries, almond milk, and chia seeds.
c. Blend until smooth and creamy.
d. Pour into a glass and enjoy.

3. **Citrus Twist**:

Ingredients:
- 2 oranges
- 1 grapefruit
- 1 lime
- 1 handful mint leaves

Procedure:
a. Peel the oranges, grapefruit, and lime.
b. Separate the segments of the oranges and grapefruit.
c. Place the citrus segments and the mint leaves in a juicer.
d. Extract the juice and pour it into a glass.
e. Garnish with a mint sprig if desired and serve.

4. **Tropical Paradise**:

Ingredients:
- 1 cup pineapple
- 1 banana
- 1 cup coconut water
- 1 tablespoon flaxseeds

Procedure:
a. Peel the pineapple and banana.
b. Cut the pineapple and banana into chunks.
c. In a blender, combine the pineapple, banana, coconut water, and flaxseeds.
d. Blend until smooth and creamy.
e. Pour into a glass and enjoy.

5. **Carrot Zinger**:

Ingredients:
- 4 carrots
- 1 apple
- 1-inch ginger
- 1 lemon

Procedure:
a. Wash and peel the carrots, apple, ginger, and lemon.
b. Cut them into pieces.
c. Put all the ingredients into a juicer and extract the juice.
d. Stir the juice well and serve chilled.

6. **Green Energy Boost**:

Ingredients:
- 2 cups kale
- 1 cucumber
- 2 green apples
- 1 lemon

Procedure:

a. Wash the kale, cucumber, green apples, and lemon.

b. Cut them into pieces.

c. Feed all the ingredients into a juicer and extract the juice.

d. Stir the juice well and serve chilled.

7. **Watermelon Cooler**:

Ingredients:
- 2 cups watermelon
- 1 cup cucumber
- 1 lime
- 1 tablespoon fresh basil

Procedure:

a. Remove the rind from the watermelon and cut it into chunks.

b. Peel the cucumber and lime.

c. Cut the cucumber into pieces.

d. In a blender, combine the watermelon, cucumber, lime juice, and fresh basil.

e. Blend until smooth and refreshing.

f. Pour into a glass and serve chilled.

8. **Beet-Berry Blend**:

Ingredients:
- 1 medium beetroot
- 1 cup strawberries
- 1 cup raspberries
- 1 cup coconut water

Procedure:
a. Wash and peel the beetroot.
b. Rinse the strawberries and raspberries.
c. In a blender, combine the beetroot, strawberries, raspberries, and coconut water.
d. Blend until smooth and vibrant.
e. Pour into a glass and enjoy.

9. **Pineapple Spinach Surprise**:

Ingredients:
- 2 cups spinach
- 1 cup pineapple
- 1 green apple
- 1 lemon

Procedure:
a. Wash the spinach, pineapple, green apple, and lemon.
b. Cut them into pieces.
c. Feed all the ingredients into a juicer and extract the juice.

d. Stir the juice well and serve chilled.

10. **Cucumber Mint Refresher**:

Ingredients:
- 1 cucumber
- 1 lime
- 1 cup mint leaves
- 1 tablespoon honey

Procedure:
a. Wash the cucumber, lime, and mint leaves.
b. Cut the cucumber into chunks.
   c. In a blender, combine the cucumber, lime juice, mint leaves, and honey.
d. Blend until well combined and refreshing.
e. Pour into a glass and serve chilled.

11. **Ginger Spice**:

Ingredients:
- 2 apples
- 1 orange
- 1-inch ginger
- 1 tablespoon turmeric

Procedure:
a. Wash the apples, orange, and ginger.
b. Cut them into pieces.
   c. Feed all the ingredients into a juicer and extract the juice.
d. Stir the juice well and serve chilled.

12. **Green Cleanse**:

Ingredients:
- 2 cups kale
- 1 cucumber
- 1 green apple
- 1 lemon
- 1 tablespoon spirulina powder

Procedure:
a. Wash the kale, cucumber, green apple, and lemon.
b. Cut them into pieces.
c. Feed all the ingredients into a juicer and extract the juice.
d. Stir in the spirulina powder until well combined.
e. Serve chilled.

13. **Berry Beet Blast**:

Ingredients:
- 1 medium beetroot
- 1 cup blueberries
- 1 cup strawberries
- 1 cup almond milk

Procedure:
a. Wash and peel the beetroot.
b. Rinse the blueberries and strawberries.
c. In a blender, combine the beetroot, blueberries, strawberries, and almond milk.

d. Blend until smooth and creamy.

e. Pour into a glass and enjoy.

14. **Citrus Carrot Crush**:

Ingredients:
- 4 carrots
- 2 oranges
- 1 lemon
- 1-inch ginger

Procedure:

a. Wash and peel the carrots, oranges, lemon, and ginger.

b. Cut them into pieces.

c. Put all the ingredients into a juicer and extract the juice.

d. Stir the juice well and serve chilled.

15. **Mango Tango**:

Ingredients:
- 2 cups mango
- 1 banana
- 1 cup coconut water
- 1 tablespoon chia seeds

Procedure:

a. Peel the mango and banana.

b. Cut them into chunks.

c. In a blender, combine the mango, banana, coconut water, and chia seeds.

d. Blend until smooth and creamy.

e. Pour into a glass and enjoy.

16. **Detox Green Tea**:

Ingredients:
- 2 cups green tea (cooled)
- 1 cup spinach
- 1 cucumber
- 1 green apple
- 1 lemon

Procedure:

a. Brew the green tea and let it cool.

b. Wash the spinach, cucumber, green apple, and lemon.

c. Cut them into pieces.

d. In a blender, combine the cooled green tea, spinach, cucumber, green apple, and lemon.

e. Blend until smooth and well combined.

f. Pour into a glass and serve chilled.

17. **Kiwi Kale Delight**:

Ingredients:
- 2 cups kale
- 2 kiwis
- 1 green apple
- 1 tablespoon flaxseeds

Procedure:

a. Wash the kale, kiwis, and green apple.

b. Cut them into pieces.

c. In a blender, combine the kale, kiwis, green apple, and flaxseeds.

d. Blend until smooth and vibrant.

e. Pour into a glass and enjoy.

18. **Pineapple Ginger Zing**:

Ingredients:
- 2 cups pineapple
- 1-inch ginger
- 1 lime
- 1 tablespoon fresh mint leaves

Procedure:

a. Peel the pineapple and ginger.

b. Cut them into pieces.

c. Juice the lime.

d. In a blender, combine the pineapple, ginger, lime juice, and fresh mint leaves.

e. Blend until smooth and energizing.

f. Pour into a glass and serve chilled.

19. **Pomegranate Berry Boost**:

Ingredients:
- 1 cup pomegranate seeds
- 1 cup blueberries
- 1 cup raspberries
- 1 cup coconut water

Procedure:

   a. Rinse the pomegranate seeds, blueberries, and raspberries.

   b. In a blender, combine the pomegranate seeds, blueberries, raspberries, and coconut water.

   c. Blend until smooth and vibrant.

   d. Pour into a glass and enjoy.

20. Watermelon Mint Refresher:

Ingredients:
- 2 cups watermelon
- 1 cup cucumber
- 1 lime
- 1 cup mint leaves

Procedure:

   a. Remove the rind from the watermelon and cut it into chunks.

   b. Peel the cucumber and lime.

   c. Cut the cucumber into pieces.

   d. In a blender, combine the watermelon, cucumber, lime juice, and mint leaves.

   e. Blend until smooth and refreshing.

   f. Pour into a glass and serve chilled.

21. Turmeric Cleanser:

Ingredients:
- 2 apples
- 1 orange
- 1-inch turmeric

- 1 tablespoon honey

Procedure:
a. Wash and cut the apples into pieces.
b. Peel and separate the orange into segments.
c. Peel the turmeric and chop it into smaller chunks.
d. Feed all the ingredients into a juicer and extract the juice.
e. Stir in the honey.
f. Serve it chilled.

22. **Green Protein Power**:

Ingredients:
- 2 cups spinach
- 1 banana
- 1 cup almond milk
- 1 tablespoon almond butter

Procedure:
a. Wash the spinach.
b. Peel and slice the banana.
c. In a blender, combine the spinach, banana, almond milk, and almond butter.
d. Blend until smooth and creamy.
e. Pour into a glass and enjoy.

23. **Lemon Ginger Blast**:

Ingredients:
- 2 apples
- 1 lemon

- 1-inch ginger
- 1 tablespoon honey

Procedure:
a. Wash and cut the apples into pieces.
b. Juice the lemon.
c. Peel and chop the ginger.
d. Feed all the ingredients into a juicer and extract the juice.
e. Stir in the honey.
f. Serve it chilled.

24. **Carrot Celery Cleanser**:

Ingredients:
- 4 carrots
- 2 stalks celery
- 1 green apple
- 1 lemon

Procedure:
a. Wash and peel the carrots.
b. Wash the celery stalks and cut them into smaller pieces.
c. Wash and cut the green apple into pieces.
d. Juice the lemon.
e. Feed all the ingredients into a juicer and extract the juice.
f. Serve it chilled.

25. **Blueberry Kale Revitalizer**:

Ingredients:
- 2 cups kale
- 1 cup blueberries
- 1 green apple
- 1 tablespoon chia seeds

Procedure:
a. Wash the kale and the blueberries.
b. Cut the green apple into pieces.
c. In a blender, combine the kale, blueberries, green apple, and chia seeds.
d. Blend until smooth and well combined.
e. Pour into a glass and enjoy.

26. **Citrus Punch**:

Ingredients:
- 2 oranges
- 1 grapefruit
- 1 lemon
- 1 tablespoon fresh mint leaves

Procedure:
a. Peel and separate the oranges and grapefruit into segments.
b. Juice the lemon.
c. Rinse the fresh mint leaves.
d. In a juicer, combine the oranges, grapefruit, lemon juice, and mint leaves.
e. Extract the juice and pour it into a glass.

f. Stir the juice well and serve it chilled.

27. **Green Hydrator**:

Ingredients:
- 2 cups spinach
- 1 cucumber
- 2 green apples
- 1 lemon
- 1 cup coconut water

Procedure:
a. Wash the spinach.
b. Wash and slice the cucumber.
c. Cut the green apples into pieces.
d. Juice the lemon.
e. In a juicer, combine the spinach, cucumber, green apples, lemon juice, and coconut water.
f. Extract the juice and pour it into a glass.
g. Stir the juice well and serve it chilled.

28. **Berry Blast Delight**:

Ingredients:
- 1 cup strawberries
- 1 cup blueberries
- 1 cup raspberries
- 1 cup almond milk
- 1 tablespoon flaxseeds

Procedure:

a. Wash the strawberries, blueberries, and raspberries.

b. In a blender, combine the berries and almond milk.

c. Blend until smooth and creamy.

d. Pour into a glass and sprinkle flaxseeds on top and Enjoy.

29. **Lemon Lime Refresher**:

Ingredients:
- 2 lemons
- 2 limes
- 1 cup cucumber
- 1 tablespoon fresh basil

Procedure:

a. Juice the lemons and limes.

b. Wash and slice the cucumber.

c. Rinse the fresh basil leaves.

d. In a juicer, combine the lemon juice, lime juice, cucumber, and fresh basil leaves.

e. Extract the juice and pour it into a glass.

f. Stir the juice well and serve it chilled.

30. **Pineapple Cucumber Cooler**:

Ingredients:
- 2 cups pineapple
- 1 cup cucumber
- 1 lime

- 1 tablespoon fresh mint leaves

Procedure:
a. Cut the pineapple into chunks.
b. Wash and slice the cucumber.
c. Juice the lime.
d. Rinse the fresh mint leaves.
e. In a juicer, combine the pineapple, cucumber, lime juice, and fresh mint leaves.
f. Extract the juice and pour it into a glass.
g. Stir the juice well and serve it chilled.

31. **Apple Celery Cleanse**:

Ingredients:
- 2 green apples
- 2 stalks celery
- 1 lemon
- 1 tablespoon honey

Procedure:
a. Wash and cut the green apples into pieces.
b. Wash the celery stalks and cut them into smaller pieces.
c. Juice the lemon.
d. In a juicer, combine the green apples, celery, and lemon juice.
e. Extract the juice and pour it into a glass.
f. Stir in the honey.
g. Serve it chilled.

32. **Spinach Detoxifier**:

Ingredients:
- 2 cups spinach
- 1 green apple
- 1 cucumber
- 1-inch ginger

Procedure:
a. Wash the spinach.
b. Cut the green apple into pieces.
c. Wash and slice the cucumber.
d. Peel and chop the ginger.
e. In a juicer, combine the spinach, green apple, cucumber, and ginger.
f. Extract the juice and pour it into a glass.
g. Stir the juice well and serve it chilled.

33. **Strawberry Watermelon Refresher**:

Ingredients:
- 2 cups watermelon
- 1 cup strawberries
- 1 lime
- 1 tablespoon chia seeds

Procedure:
a. Cut the watermelon into chunks.
b. Wash the strawberries.
c. Juice the lime.

d. In a juicer, combine the watermelon, strawberries, lime juice, and chia seeds.
e. Extract the juice and pour it into a glass.
f. Stir the juice well and serve it chilled.

34. **Mango Passion**:

Ingredients:
- 2 cups mango
- 1 banana
- 1 cup coconut water
- 1 tablespoon flaxseeds

Procedure:
a. Peel and chop the mango.
b. Peel and slice the banana.
c. In a blender, combine the mango, banana, coconut water, and flaxseeds.
d. Blend until smooth and creamy.
e. Pour into a glass and enjoy.

35. **Cucumber Lemon Splash**:

Ingredients:
- 1 cucumber
- 2 lemons
- 1 cup mint leaves
- 1 tablespoon honey

Procedure:
a. Wash and slice the cucumber.
b. Juice the lemons.

c. Rinse the mint leaves.

d. In a blender, combine the cucumber slices, lemon juice, mint leaves, and honey.

e. Blend until well combined and refreshing.

f. Serve chilled after pouring into a glass.

Enjoy these delicious and nutritious recipes as part of your weight loss journey! Remember to consult with a healthcare professional or registered dietitian before making significant changes to your diet, especially if you have any underlying health conditions.

CHAPTER THREE

DETOXIFICATION THROUGH JUICING

Detoxification through juicing has gained significant popularity in recent years as a natural and effective way to cleanse the body and promote overall well-being. This approach involves consuming freshly made juices from a variety of fruits, vegetables, and herbs, which are believed to help eliminate toxins and support the body's natural detoxification processes. In this article, we will explore the significance of bodily detoxification and delve into some detoxifying ingredients and their benefits.

The Significance of Bodily Detoxification

Detoxification is the process by which the body eliminates harmful substances, often referred to as toxins, that accumulate due to various factors such as poor diet, environmental pollutants, and stress. These toxins can overload our organs, particularly the liver, kidneys, and colon, making it difficult for them to function optimally. Consequently, this can lead to a range of health issues, including fatigue, digestive problems, skin disorders, and a weakened immune system.

Detoxification is vital because it helps the body restore balance and improve its natural detox mechanisms. By eliminating toxins, the body can better absorb essential nutrients, enhance cellular function, and support various bodily systems. Moreover, detoxification can contribute to increased energy levels, improved digestion, clearer skin, mental clarity, and overall vitality.

Detoxifying Ingredients and Their Benefits

1. Leafy Greens: Green vegetables such as kale, spinach, and Swiss chard are rich in chlorophyll, a powerful detoxifier that aids in the elimination of toxins from the bloodstream. These greens also provide essential vitamins, minerals, and antioxidants that support liver function and promote overall health.

2. Citrus Fruits: Lemons, limes, and grapefruits are excellent sources of vitamin C and antioxidants. They help stimulate the production of enzymes that support liver detoxification and promote the removal of toxins from the body. Citrus fruits also have alkalizing properties, which can help restore the body's pH balance.

3. Ginger: Known for its anti-inflammatory and digestive benefits, ginger can aid in the

detoxification process. It helps stimulate digestion, enhances circulation, and supports liver function. Ginger also possesses antioxidant properties that protect against free radicals and oxidative stress.

4. Beetroot: This vibrant root vegetable is a potent detoxifier and blood purifier. Beetroot contains a compound called betaine, which supports liver function and aids in the elimination of toxins. Additionally, beetroot is rich in antioxidants, fiber, and vitamins that promote overall health.

5. Turmeric: A spice widely used in traditional medicine, turmeric contains curcumin, a compound with powerful anti-inflammatory and antioxidant properties. Turmeric can support liver detoxification, reduce inflammation, and promote overall well-being.

6. Cucumber: Cucumbers are excellent hydrators and natural diuretics, which help flush out toxins from the body. They are also low in calories and high in fiber, making them beneficial for maintaining a healthy weight and supporting digestion.

7. Wheatgrass: This young grass is packed with nutrients and chlorophyll, making it a potent detoxifying ingredient. Wheatgrass can help eliminate toxins, boost energy levels, support liver function, and improve digestion.

35 revitalizing recipes for detoxification

Here's a comprehensive guide to the ingredients and procedures for juicing recipes for detoxification:

1. Green Machine Detox:

Ingredients:
- 2 cups spinach
- 1 cucumber
- 2 green apples
- 1 lemon, peeled
- 1-inch piece of ginger

Procedure:
- Wash the spinach, cucumber, green apples, lemon, and ginger.
- Cut them into pieces.
- Feed all the ingredients into a juicer and extract the juice.
- Stir the juice well and serve it chilled.

2. Beet and Carrot Cleanser:

Ingredients:
- 2 medium beets
- 3 carrots
- 1 orange, peeled
- 1-inch piece of turmeric

Procedure:
- Clean and peel the carrots and beets..
- Rinse the orange and turmeric.
- Feed all the ingredients into a juicer and extract the juice.
- Stir the juice well and serve it chilled.

3. **Citrus Blast**:

Ingredients:
- 2 oranges, peeled
- 1 grapefruit, peeled
- 2 lemons, peeled
- 1 lime, peeled
- 1 tablespoon fresh mint leaves

Procedure:
- Peel the oranges, grapefruit, lemons, and lime.
- Place the citrus fruits and fresh mint leaves in a juicer.
- Extract the juice and pour it into a glass.
- Stir the juice well and serve it chilled.

4. **Cucumber Celery Refresher**:

Ingredients:
- 2 cucumbers
- 4 celery stalks
- 1 green apple
- 1 lemon, peeled

Procedure:
- Wash the cucumbers, celery stalks, green apple, and lemon.
- Cut them into pieces.
- Put all the ingredients into a juicer and extract the juice.
- Stir the juice well and serve it chilled.

5. **Tropical Detox Delight**:

Ingredients:
- 1 cup pineapple chunks
- 1 cup mango chunks
- 1 banana
- 1 orange, peeled
- 1 tablespoon chia seeds

Procedure:
- Peel and chop the pineapple, mango, and orange.
- Peel and slice the banana.
- In a blender, combine all the fruits with chia seeds.
- Blend until smooth and creamy.
- Pour into a glass and enjoy.

6. **Lemon Ginger Detoxifier**:

Ingredients:
- 2 lemons, peeled
- 1 cucumber
- 1-inch piece of ginger
- 1 tablespoon honey (optional)

Procedure:
- Wash the lemons, cucumber, and ginger.
- Cut them into pieces.
- Feed all the ingredients into a juicer and extract the juice.
- Stir in honey if desired.
- Serve it chilled.

7. Watermelon Mint Cooler:

Ingredients:
- 3 cups watermelon chunks
- 1 cucumber
- 1 lime, peeled
- 10 fresh mint leaves

Procedure:
- Remove the rind from the watermelon and cut it into chunks.
- Wash the cucumber, lime, and mint leaves.
- In a blender, combine the watermelon, cucumber, lime juice, and mint leaves.
- Blend until smooth and refreshing.
- Serve chilled after pouring into a glass.

8. Pineapple Kale Cleanse:

Ingredients:
- 2 cups kale
- 1 cup pineapple chunks
- 1 green apple

- 1 lemon, peeled

Procedure:
- Wash the kale, pineapple, green apple, and lemon.
- Cut them into pieces.
- Feed all the ingredients into a juicer and extract the juice.
- Stir the juice well and serve it chilled.

9. **Carrot Ginger Zinger**:

Ingredients:
- 4 carrots
- 1 apple
- 1-inch piece of ginger

Procedure:
- Wash and peel the carrots, apple, and ginger.
- Juice the lemon.
- Feed all the ingredients into a juicer and extract the juice.
- Stir in the lemon juice.
- Serve it chilled.

10. **Berry Antioxidant Boost**:

Ingredients:
- 1 cup strawberries
- 1 cup blueberries
- 1 cup raspberries
- 1 cup almond milk

Procedure:
- Wash the strawberries, blueberries, and raspberries.
- In a blender, combine the berries with almond milk.
- Blend until smooth and creamy.
- Pour into a glass and enjoy.

11. **Green Detox Elixir**:

Ingredients:
- 2 cups spinach
- 1 cucumber
- 2 green apples
- 1 lemon, peeled
- 1-inch piece of ginger

Procedure:
- Wash the spinach, cucumber, green apples, lemon, and ginger.
- Cut them into pieces.
- Feed all the ingredients into a juicer and extract the juice.
- Stir the juice well and serve it chilled.

12. **Detoxifying Beetroot Blend**:

Ingredients:
- 2 medium beets
- 2 carrots
- 1 apple

- 1 orange, peeled

Procedure:
- Wash and peel the beets, carrots, and apple.
- Peel the orange.
- Feed all the ingredients into a juicer and extract the juice.
- Stir the juice well and serve it chilled.

13. Citrus Beet Cleanser:

Ingredients:
- 1 medium beet
- 2 oranges, peeled
- 1 grapefruit, peeled
- 1 tablespoon fresh mint leaves

Procedure:
- Wash and peel the beet and citrus fruits.
- Place them in a juicer along with fresh mint leaves.
- Extract the juice and pour it into a glass.
- Stir the juice well and serve it chilled.

14. Cucumber Basil Refresher:

Ingredients:
- 2 cucumbers
- 1 cup fresh basil leaves
- 1 lime, peeled
- 1 tablespoon honey (optional)

Procedure:
- Wash the cucumbers and lime.
- Rinse the fresh basil leaves.
- In a blender, combine the cucumbers, lime juice, basil leaves, and honey.
- Blend until well combined and refreshing.
- Serve chilled after pouring into a glass.

15. **Mango Papaya Detox Blast**:

Ingredients:
- 1 cup mango chunks
- 1 cup papaya chunks
- 1 orange, peeled
- 1 tablespoon chia seeds

Procedure:
- Peel and chop the mango and papaya.
- Peel and slice the orange.
- In a blender, combine all the fruits with chia seeds.
- Blend until smooth and creamy.
- Pour into a glass and enjoy.

16. **Lemon Turmeric Tonic**:

Ingredients:
- 2 lemons, peeled
- 1 cucumber
- 1-inch piece of turmeric
- 1 tablespoon honey (optional)

Procedure:
- Wash the lemons, cucumber, and turmeric.
- Cut them into pieces.
- Feed all the ingredients into a juicer and extract the juice.
- Stir in honey if desired.
- Serve it chilled.

17. **Watermelon Berry Cleanser**:

Ingredients:
- 2 cups watermelon chunks
- 1 cup of mixed berries, which include strawberries, blueberries, and raspberries
- 1 lime, peeled
- 10 fresh mint leaves

Procedure:
- Remove the rind from the watermelon and cut it into chunks.
- Wash the mixed berries and lime.
- Rinse the fresh mint leaves.
- In a blender, combine the watermelon, mixed berries, lime juice, and mint leaves.
- Blend until smooth and refreshing.
- Serve chilled after pouring into a glass.

18. **Kale Pineapple Detox**:

Ingredients:
- 2 cups kale
- 1 cup pineapple chunks

- 1 green apple
- 1 lemon, peeled

Procedure:
- Wash the kale, pineapple, green apple, and lemon.
- Cut them into pieces.
- Feed all the ingredients into a juicer and extract the juice.
- Stir the juice well and serve it chilled.

19. **Carrot Apple Ginger Cleanse**:

Ingredients:
- 4 carrots
- 2 green apples
- 1-inch piece of ginger
- 1 tablespoon lemon juice

Procedure:
- Wash and peel the carrots, green apples, and ginger.
- Juice the lemon.
- Feed all the ingredients into a juicer and extract the juice.
- Stir in the lemon juice.
- Serve it chilled.

20. **Mixed Berry Powerhouse**:

Ingredients:
- 1 cup strawberries

- 1 cup blueberries
- 1 cup raspberries
- 1 cup coconut water

Procedure:
- Wash the strawberries, blueberries, and raspberries.
- In a blender, combine the berries with coconut water.
- Blend until smooth and creamy.
- Pour into a glass and enjoy.

21. **Green Revitalizer**:

Ingredients:
- 2 cups spinach
- 1 cucumber
- 2 green apples
- 1 lemon, peeled
- 1-inch piece of ginger

Procedure:
- Wash the spinach, cucumber, green apples, lemon, and ginger.
- Cut them into pieces.
- Feed all the ingredients into a juicer and extract the juice.
- Stir the juice well and serve it chilled.

22. Beetroot Citrus Refresher:

Ingredients:
- 2 medium beets
- 2 oranges, peeled
- 1 grapefruit, peeled
- 1 tablespoon fresh mint leaves

Procedure:
- Wash and peel the beets and citrus fruits.
- Place them in a juicer along with fresh mint leaves.
- Extract the juice and pour it into a glass.
- Stir the juice well and serve it chilled.

23. Cucumber Mint Cooler:

Ingredients:
- 2 cucumbers
- 1 cup fresh mint leaves
- 1 lime, peeled
- 1 tablespoon honey (optional)

Procedure:
- Wash the cucumbers and lime.
- Rinse the fresh mint leaves.
- In a blender, combine the cucumbers, lime juice, mint leaves, and honey.
- Blend until well combined and refreshing.
- Serve chilled after pouring into a glass.

24. **Papaya Kiwi Cleanse**:

Ingredients:
- 1 cup papaya chunks
- 1 kiwi, peeled
- 1 orange, peeled
- 1 tablespoon chia seeds

Procedure:
- Peel and chop the papaya.
- Peel and cut the kiwi and orange into slices.
- In a blender, combine all the fruits with chia seeds.
- Blend until smooth and creamy.
- Pour into a glass and enjoy.

25. **Lemon Cayenne Detox Shot**:

Ingredients:
- Juice of 2 lemons
- 1/4 teaspoon cayenne pepper
- 1 teaspoon maple syrup (optional)
- 1 cup filtered water

Procedure:
- Juice the lemons.
- Stir in cayenne pepper and maple syrup (if using) with filtered water.
- Pour the mixture into a shot glass and consume it quickly.

26. **Watermelon Cucumber Detox**:

Ingredients:
- 2 cups watermelon chunks
- 1 cucumber
- 1 lime, peeled
- 10 fresh mint leaves

Procedure:
- Remove the rind from the watermelon and cut it into chunks.
- Wash the cucumber, lime, and mint leaves.
- Combine the watermelon, cucumber, lime juice, and mint leaves in a blender.
- Blend until smooth and refreshing.
- Serve chilled after pouring into a glass.

27. **Spinach Pineapple Mint Blend**:

Ingredients:
- 2 cups spinach
- 1 cup pineapple chunks
- 1 green apple
- 1 lemon, peeled
- 5 fresh mint leaves

Procedure:
- Wash the spinach, pineapple, green apple, lemon, and mint leaves.
- Cut them into pieces.
- Feed all the ingredients into a juicer and extract the juice.

- Stir the juice well and serve it chilled.

28. **Gingered Carrot Apple Cleanse**:

Ingredients:
- 4 carrots
- 1 green apple
- 1-inch piece of ginger
- 1 tablespoon lemon juice

Procedure:
- Wash and peel the carrots, green apple, and ginger.
- Juice the lemon.
- Feed all the ingredients into a juicer and extract the juice.
- Stir in the lemon juice.
- Serve it chilled.

29. **Blueberry Pomegranate Antioxidant Juice:**

Ingredients:
- 1 cup blueberries
- 1/2 cup pomegranate seeds
- 1 cup coconut water

Procedure:
- Wash the blueberries.
- In a blender, combine the blueberries, pomegranate seeds, and coconut water.
- Blend until smooth and well combined.

- Pour into a glass and enjoy.

30. **Kale Celery Detoxifier**:

Ingredients:
- 2 cups kale
- 4 celery stalks
- 1 green apple
- 1 lemon, peeled

Procedure:
- Wash the kale, celery stalks, green apple, and lemon.
- Cut them into pieces.
- Feed all the ingredients into a juicer and extract the juice.
- Stir the juice well and serve it chilled.

31. **Green Detox Elixir**:

Ingredients:
- 2 cups spinach
- 1 cucumber
- 2 green apples
- 1 lemon, peeled
- 1-inch piece of ginger

Procedure:
- Wash the spinach, cucumber, green apples, lemon, and ginger.
- Cut them into pieces.

- Feed all the ingredients into a juicer and extract the juice.
- Stir the juice well and serve it chilled.

32. **Beetroot Orange Refresher**:

Ingredients:
- 2 medium beets
- 3 oranges, peeled
- 1 tablespoon fresh mint leaves

Procedure:
- Wash and peel the beets and oranges.
- Place them in a juicer along with fresh mint leaves.
- Extract the juice and pour it into a glass.
- Stir the juice well and serve it chilled.

33. **Cucumber Lemon Basil Cooler**:

Ingredients:
- 2 cucumbers
- 1 lemon, peeled
- 1 cup fresh basil leaves
- 1 tablespoon honey (optional)

Procedure:
- Wash the cucumbers and lemon.
- Rinse the fresh basil leaves.
- In a blender, combine the cucumbers, lemon juice, basil leaves, and honey.
- Blend until well combined and refreshing.

- Serve chilled after pouring into a glass.

34. **Mango Banana Detox Smoothie**:

Ingredients:
- 1 cup mango chunks
- 1 banana
- 1 orange, peeled
- 1 tablespoon chia seeds

Procedure:
- Peel and chop the mango.
- The banana and orange should be peeled and sliced.
-- In a blender, combine all the fruits with chia seeds.
- Blend until smooth and creamy.
- Pour into a glass and enjoy.

35. **Lemon Ginger Mint Cleanser**:

Ingredients:
- 2 lemons, peeled
- 1 cucumber
- 1-inch piece of ginger
- 1 tablespoon fresh mint leaves

Procedure:
- Wash the lemons, cucumber, and ginger.
- Rinse the fresh mint leaves.
- Cut the lemons, cucumber, and ginger into pieces.

- In a blender, combine the lemons, cucumber, ginger, and fresh mint leaves.
- Blend until well combined.
- Serve chilled after pouring into a glass.

These 35 juicing recipes offer a wide variety of delicious and refreshing options for detoxification. They are packed with nutrients and antioxidants that can help cleanse your body and boost your overall well-being. Whether you prefer green juices, citrus blends, or fruity concoctions, there is something for everyone on this list. Enjoy these recipes as part of a balanced diet and a healthy lifestyle. Cheers to good health!

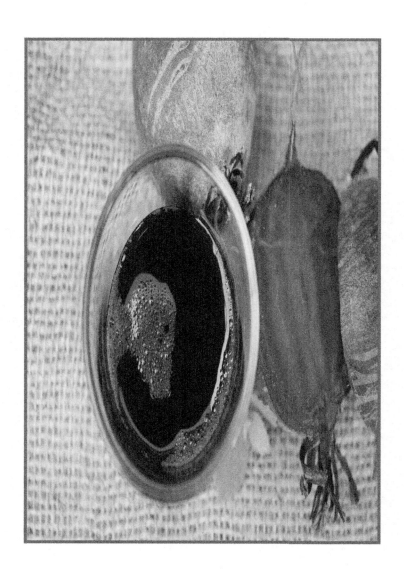

CHAPTER FOUR

PREVENTING AGING WITH JUICING

As we age, our bodies undergo various physiological changes that can impact our overall health and well-being. The aging process is influenced by both intrinsic factors (such as genetics) and extrinsic factors (such as lifestyle choices and environmental factors). While aging is a natural and inevitable process, there are steps we can take to slow down the effects of aging and promote healthy aging.

One effective approach to promoting healthy aging is through proper nutrition, and juicing can play a significant role in this regard. Juicing involves extracting the juice from fruits and vegetables, providing a concentrated dose of essential nutrients, antioxidants, and phytochemicals that can support overall health and help prevent or slow down the aging process.

Antioxidants and their Role in Preventing Aging

Antioxidants are compounds found in various fruits, vegetables, and other plant-based foods that help protect our cells from damage caused by free radicals. Free radicals are unstable molecules that are generated as byproducts of normal cellular metabolism and are also produced in response to factors such as pollution, smoking, and excessive sun exposure. These free radicals can cause oxidative stress, leading to cellular damage and contributing to the aging process.

The body has its own defense mechanisms to neutralize free radicals, but these may become less effective with age. This is where antioxidants come into play. Antioxidants help neutralize free radicals, reducing oxidative stress and preventing or minimizing cellular damage. By including antioxidant-rich foods in our diet, such as those commonly found in juicing recipes, we can enhance our body's natural defense against aging and support overall health.

Benefits of Antioxidant-Rich Juices

Juicing provides an excellent way to increase your intake of antioxidants and other beneficial compounds. Here are some key benefits of consuming antioxidant-rich juices:

1. Reduced Oxidative Stress: Antioxidants help combat oxidative stress by neutralizing free radicals, reducing cellular damage, and promoting overall cellular health.

2. Skin Health: Aging is often associated with changes in the skin, including wrinkles, dryness, and loss of elasticity. Antioxidant-rich juices can provide essential nutrients that support skin health, helping to maintain a youthful appearance and reducing the signs of aging.

3. Brain Health: Oxidative stress and inflammation have been linked to age-related cognitive decline and neurodegenerative diseases. Antioxidant-rich juices can help reduce oxidative stress in the brain, supporting cognitive function and promoting brain health as we age.

4. Heart Health: The aging process is associated with an increased risk of cardiovascular diseases. Antioxidant-rich juices, particularly those containing fruits and vegetables rich in flavonoids and polyphenols, can help protect against heart disease by reducing inflammation, supporting healthy blood vessels, and improving cardiovascular function.

5. Eye Health: Age-related macular degeneration (AMD) is a common eye condition that can cause vision loss in older adults. Antioxidant-rich juices, particularly those containing dark leafy greens and colorful fruits and vegetables, are rich in nutrients such as lutein and zeaxanthin that can help protect against AMD and maintain healthy vision.

Incorporating Antioxidant-Rich Juices into Your Diet

To maximize the anti-aging benefits of juicing, consider incorporating the following antioxidant-rich ingredients into your juice recipes:

- Berries: Blueberries, strawberries, raspberries, and blackberries are packed with antioxidants and other beneficial compounds that help fight free radicals.

- Dark Leafy Greens: Spinach, kale, Swiss chard, and collard greens are excellent sources of antioxidants, vitamins, and minerals that support overall health and combat the aging process.

- Citrus Fruits: Oranges, lemons, grapefruits, and limes are rich in vitamin C, a potent antioxidant that supports collagen production, skin health, and immune function.

- Carrots: Carrots are not only rich in antioxidants but also contain beta-carotene, which the body converts into vitamin A.For healthy skin and eyesight, vitamin A is necessary.

- Tomatoes: Tomatoes contain lycopene, a powerful antioxidant known for its anti-aging properties and its potential to protect against types of cancer.

- Green Tea: Green tea is a rich source of catechins, which are potent antioxidants that help fight inflammation and protect against age-related diseases.

When juicing, aim for a variety of antioxidant-rich ingredients to maximize the benefits. Remember to consume your juices immediately to ensure optimal freshness and nutrient content. Consider incorporating juicing into a balanced diet that includes whole foods, lean proteins, healthy fats, and regular exercise for comprehensive anti-aging benefits.

35 anti-aging recipes to promote youthful vitality

Here's a comprehensive guide to the ingredients and procedures for delicious recipes for preventing aging to promote youthful vitality:

1. Green Glow:

Ingredients:
- 2 cups spinach
- 1 cucumber
- 1 green apple

- 1/2 lemon (peeled)
- 1-inch piece of ginger

Procedure:
1. Wash the spinach thoroughly and chop it if necessary.
2. Peel the cucumber and cut it into chunks.
3. Core the green apple and cut it into pieces.
4. Juice the spinach, cucumber, green apple, peeled lemon, and ginger together.
5. Stir the juice well and serve it fresh.

2. Carrot Cleanser:

Ingredients:
- 4 carrots
- 1 beetroot (peeled)
- 1 orange (peeled)
- 1-inch piece of turmeric

Procedure:
1. Carrots, beets, and oranges should be washed and peeled.
2. Cut the carrots and beetroot into smaller pieces.
3. Juice the carrots, beetroot, peeled orange, and turmeric together.
4. Mix well and enjoy the juice immediately.

3. **Berry Blast**:

Ingredients:
- 1 cup of blueberries, strawberries, and raspberries mixed together.
- 1 banana
- 1 cup almond milk
- 1 tablespoon chia seeds

Procedure:
1. Rinse the mixed berries and remove any stems or leaves.
2. Peel the banana and break it into chunks.
3. Combine the mixed berries, banana, almond milk, and chia seeds in a blender.
4. Blend until smooth and creamy.
5. Pour the mixture into a glass and serve chilled.

4. **Tropical Delight**:

Ingredients:
- 1 cup pineapple
- 1 orange (peeled)
- 1 kiwi (peeled)
- 1/2 cup coconut water

Procedure:
1. Cut the pineapple, peeled orange, and peeled kiwi into chunks.

2. Add the pineapple, orange, kiwi, and coconut water to a blender.
3. Blend until smooth and well combined.
4. Pour into a glass and enjoy the tropical flavors.

5. **Antioxidant Elixir**:

Ingredients:
- 1 cup kale
- 1 cup spinach
- 1 cup grapes
- 1 green apple
- 1/2 lime (peeled)

Procedure:
1. Wash the kale and spinach thoroughly.
2. Core the green apple and cut it into pieces.
3. Juice the kale, spinach, grapes, green apple, and peeled lime together.
4. Stir well and serve the elixir fresh.

6. **Citrus Zing**:

Ingredients:
- 2 oranges (peeled)
- 1 grapefruit (peeled)
- 1 lemon (peeled)
- 1-inch piece of ginger

Procedure:
1. Peel the oranges, grapefruit, and lemon.
2. Slice the peeled fruits into smaller pieces.

3. Juice the oranges, grapefruit, lemon, and ginger together.
4. Mix the juice thoroughly and enjoy its refreshing zing.

7. **Super Skin Booster**:

Ingredients:
- 2 carrots
- 1 sweet potato
- 1 bell pepper (any color)
- 1 apple
- 1/2 lemon (peeled)

Procedure:
1. Wash and peel the carrots, sweet potato, and lemon.
2. Cut the carrots, sweet potato, bell pepper, and apple into smaller pieces.
3. Juice the carrots, sweet potato, bell pepper, apple, and peeled lemon together.
4. Stir the juice well and drink it for a super skin boost.

8. **Cucumber Cooler**:

Ingredients:
- 2 cucumbers
- 1 cup watermelon
- 1/2 lime (peeled)
- Fresh mint leaves

Procedure:
1. Peel the cucumbers and cut them into chunks.
2. Chop the watermelon into smaller pieces.
3. Juice the cucumbers, watermelon, peeled lime, and a handful of fresh mint leaves together.
4. Stir well and serve chilled for a refreshing and cooling effect.

9. **Pomegranate Power**:

Ingredients:
- 1 cup pomegranate seeds
- 1 cup spinach
- 1 apple
- 1/2 cucumber
- 1-inch piece of ginger

Procedure:
1. Extract the pomegranate seeds from the pomegranate fruit.
2. Wash the spinach thoroughly.
3. Core the apple and cut it into pieces.
4. Peel the cucumber and cut it into chunks.
5. Juice the pomegranate seeds, spinach, apple, cucumber, and ginger together.
6. Mix the juice well and enjoy its powerful antioxidant properties.

10. **Pineapple Paradise**:

Ingredients:
- 2 cups pineapple

- 1 orange (peeled)
- 1/2 lemon (peeled)
- 1/2 lime (peeled)

Procedure:
1. Cut the pineapple into chunks.
2. Peel the orange, lemon, and lime.
3. Slice the peeled fruits into smaller pieces.
4. Juice the pineapple, peeled orange, peeled lemon, and peeled lime together.
5. Stir the juice well and savor the tropical paradise flavors.

11. **Beet-iful Glow**:

Ingredients:
- 2 beetroots (peeled)
- 2 carrots
- 1 apple
- 1-inch piece of ginger

Procedure:
1. Wash and peel the beetroots, carrots, and ginger.
2. Cut the beetroots, carrots, apple, and ginger into smaller pieces.
3. Juice the beetroots, carrots, apple, and ginger together.
4. Mix well and enjoy the juice for its beautifying properties.

12. **Goji Berry Boost**:

Ingredients:
- 1 cup goji berries
- 1 cup kale
- 1 orange (peeled)
- 1 banana
- 1/2 cup coconut water

Procedure:
1. Rinse the goji berries.
2. Wash the kale thoroughly.
3. Peel the orange and banana.
4. Combine the goji berries, kale, peeled orange, peeled banana, and coconut water in a blender.
5. Blend until smooth and creamy.
6. Pour the mixture into a glass and drink it for a revitalizing boost.

13. **Mango Magic**:

Ingredients:
- 2 cups mango
- 1 cup spinach
- 1 orange (peeled)
- 1/2 lime (peeled)

Procedure:
1. Cut the mango into chunks.
2. Wash the spinach thoroughly.
3. Peel the orange and lime.
4. Slice the peeled fruits into smaller pieces.

5. Juice the mango, spinach, peeled orange, and peeled lime together.
6. Stir the juice well and enjoy its magical taste.

14. **Blueberry Bliss**:

Ingredients:
- 1 cup blueberries
- 1 cup almond milk
- 1 banana
- 1 tablespoon flaxseed

Procedure:
1. Rinse the blueberries and remove any stems or leaves.
2. Peel the banana and break it into chunks.
3. Combine the blueberries, almond milk, peeled banana, and flaxseed in a blender.
4. Blend until smooth and creamy.
5. Pour the mixture into a glass and savor the blissful blueberry flavor.

15. **Turmeric Tonic**:

Ingredients:
- 2 cups coconut water
- 1 tablespoon turmeric powder
- 1/2 lemon (peeled)
- 1-inch piece of ginger
- Pinch of black pepper

Procedure:
1. In a blender, combine the coconut water, turmeric powder, peeled lemon, peeled ginger, and a pinch of black pepper.
2. Blend until well combined and smooth.
3. Pour the mixture into a glass and enjoy the rejuvenating and anti-inflammatory benefits of this turmeric tonic.

16. **Kale Kickstart**:

Ingredients:
- 2 cups kale
- 1 green apple
- 1 cucumber
- 1/2 lemon (peeled)
- 1-inch piece of ginger

Procedure:
1. Wash the kale thoroughly.
2. Core the green apple and cut it into pieces.
3. Peel the cucumber and then chop it up.
4. Juice the kale, green apple, cucumber, peeled lemon, and ginger together.
5. Stir well and start your day with this refreshing and nutritious kale kickstart.

17. **Orange Radiance**:

Ingredients:
- 4 oranges (peeled)
- 2 carrots

- 1-inch piece of turmeric

Procedure:
1. Peel the oranges and remove any seeds.
2. Wash and peel the carrots.
3. Cut the oranges and carrots into smaller pieces.
4. Juice the oranges, carrots, and turmeric together.
5. Mix well and enjoy the radiant flavors of this orange elixir.

18. **Spinach Supreme**:

Ingredients:
- 2 cups spinach
- 1 green apple
- 1 cucumber
- 1/2 lime (peeled)
- Handful of fresh parsley

Procedure:
1. Wash the spinach thoroughly.
2. Core the green apple and cut it into pieces.
3. Peel the cucumber and then chop it up.
4. Juice the spinach, green apple, cucumber, peeled lime, and fresh parsley together.
5. Stir the juice well and savor the supreme taste of spinach and parsley.

19. **Carrot Ginger Refresher**:

Ingredients:
- 4 carrots

- 1 green apple
- 1-inch piece of ginger
- 1/2 lemon (peeled)

Procedure:
1. Wash and peel the carrots, ginger, and lemon.
2. Cut the carrots and green apple into smaller pieces.
3. Juice the carrots, green apple, ginger, and peeled lemon together.
4. Mix well and enjoy the refreshing and tangy flavor of this carrot ginger refresher.

20. **Raspberry Revitalizer**:

Ingredients:
- 1 cup raspberries
- 1 cup almond milk
- 1 banana
- 1 tablespoon honey

Procedure:
1. Rinse the raspberries and remove any stems or leaves.
2. Peel the banana and break it into chunks.
3. Combine the raspberries, almond milk, peeled banana, and honey in a blender.
4. Blend until smooth and creamy.
5. Pour the mixture into a glass and revitalize yourself with the sweet and tangy taste of raspberries.

21. **Watermelon Wonder**:

Ingredients:
- 2 cups watermelon
- 1 cup cucumber
- 1/2 lime (peeled)
- Fresh mint leaves

Procedure:
1. Cut the watermelon into chunks, removing any seeds if necessary.
2. Peel the cucumber and cut it into chunks.
3. Juice the watermelon, cucumber, peeled lime, and a handful of fresh mint leaves together.
4. Stir well and enjoy the refreshing and hydrating properties of this watermelon wonder.

22. **Kiwi Green**:

Ingredients:
- 2 kiwis (peeled)
- 1 cup spinach
- 1 green apple
- 1/2 lemon (peeled)

Procedure:
1. Wash the spinach thoroughly.
2. Core the green apple and cut it into pieces.
3. Peel the kiwis and cut them into chunks.

4. Juice the kiwis, spinach, green apple, and peeled lemon together.
5. Mix the juice well and enjoy the green goodness of this kiwi delight.

23. **Ginger Lemonade**:

Ingredients:
- 2 lemons (peeled)
- 1-inch piece of ginger
- 2 cups water
- 1 tablespoon honey

Procedure:
1. Peel the lemons and slice them into smaller pieces.
2. Peel the ginger and chop it into smaller chunks.
3. In a blender, combine the peeled lemons, ginger, water, and honey.
4. Blend until well combined.
5. Pour the mixture into a glass and enjoy the zesty and refreshing taste of ginger lemonade.

24. **Grape Antioxidant Blast**:

Ingredients:
- 2 cups grapes
- 1 cup kale
- 1 green apple
- 1/2 cucumber

Procedure:
1. Rinse the grapes and remove any stems.
2. Wash the kale thoroughly.
3. Core the green apple and cut it into pieces.
4. Peel the cucumber and cut it into chunks.
5. Juice the grapes, kale, green apple, and cucumber together.
6. Stir well and indulge in the antioxidant blast of this grape-infused juice.

25. Celery Soother:

Ingredients:
- 4 celery stalks
- 1 cucumber
- 1 green apple
- 1/2 lemon (peeled)
- Handful of fresh cilantro

Procedure:
1. Wash the celery stalks and cucumber.
2. Cut the celery stalks and cucumber into smaller pieces.
3. Core the green apple and cut it into pieces.
4. Juice the celery stalks, cucumber, green apple, peeled lemon, and fresh cilantro together.
5. Mix well and enjoy the soothing and refreshing properties of this celery-based juice.

26. **Minty Melon**:

Ingredients:
- 2 cups cantaloupe
- 1 cup honeydew melon
- Fresh mint leaves

Procedure:
1. Cut the cantaloupe and honeydew melon into chunks, removing any seeds if necessary.
2. Add the melon chunks and a handful of fresh mint leaves to a blender.
3. Blend until smooth and well combined.
4. Pour the mixture into a glass and savor the minty freshness of this melon delight.

27. **Apple Carrot Cleanse**:

Ingredients:
- 2 green apples
- 2 carrots
- 1/2 lemon (peeled)
- 1-inch piece of ginger

Procedure:
1. Wash and core the green apples.
2. Wash and peel the carrots, lemon, and ginger.
3. Cut the green apples, carrots, peeled lemon, and peeled ginger into smaller pieces.

4. Juice the green apples, carrots, peeled lemon, and peeled ginger together.
5. Mix well and enjoy the cleansing and invigorating taste of this apple carrot blend.

28. Peachy Glow:

Ingredients:
- 2 peaches
- 1 cup spinach
- 1 orange (peeled)
- 1/2 lime (peeled)

Procedure:
1. Wash the spinach thoroughly.
2. Peel the peaches and remove the pits.
3. Peel the orange and lime.
4. Slice the peeled fruits into smaller pieces.
5. Juice the peaches, spinach, peeled orange, and peeled lime together.
6. Stir the juice well and savor the peachy goodness of this refreshing blend.

29. Cabbage Refresher:

Ingredients:
- 2 cups cabbage
- 1 green apple
- 1 cucumber
- 1/2 lemon (peeled)

Procedure:

1. Wash the cabbage thoroughly and cut it into smaller pieces.

2. Core the green apple and cut it into pieces.

3. Peel the cucumber and then chop it up.

4. Juice the cabbage, green apple, cucumber, and peeled lemon together.

5. Mix well and enjoy the refreshing and rejuvenating properties of this cabbage refresher.

30. **Cranberry Detox**:

Ingredients:
- 1 cup cranberries
- 2 carrots
- 1 green apple
- 1/2 lemon (peeled)

Procedure:

1. Rinse the cranberries and remove any stems.

2. Wash and peel the carrots and lemon.

3. Core the green apple and cut it into pieces.

4. Juice the cranberries, carrots, green apple, and peeled lemon together.

5. Stir well and indulge in the detoxifying and tart flavors of this cranberry-infused juice.

31. **Blackberry Beauty**:

Ingredients:
- 1 cup blackberries

- 1 cup almond milk
- 1 banana
- 1 tablespoon almond butter

Procedure:
1. Remove any stems from the blackberries and rinse them.
2. Peel the banana and break it into chunks.
3. Combine the blackberries, almond milk, peeled banana, and almond butter in a blender.
4. Blend until smooth and creamy.
5. Pour the mixture into a glass and enjoy the beauty-boosting benefits of blackberries.

32. **Pear Perfection**:

Ingredients:
- 2 pears
- 1 cup spinach
- 1 green apple
- 1/2 lemon (peeled)

Procedure:
1. Wash the spinach thoroughly.
2. Core the pears and cut them into pieces.
3. Core the green apple and cut it into pieces.
4. Peel the lemon.
5. Juice the pears, spinach, green apple, and peeled lemon together.
6. Mix well and enjoy the perfection of this pear-based juice.

33. **Tomato Time**:

Ingredients:
- 2 tomatoes
- 1 cup spinach
- 1 cucumber
- 1/2 lime (peeled)

Procedure:
1. Wash the tomatoes and spinach thoroughly.
2. Peel the cucumber and cut it into chunks.
3. Juice the tomatoes, spinach, cucumber, and peeled lime together.
4. Stir well and enjoy the fresh and tangy taste of this tomato-infused juice.

34. **Lemon Berry Detox**:

Ingredients:
- 1 cup of blueberries, strawberries, and raspberries mixed together
- 1/2 lemon (peeled)
- 2 cups water
- 1 tablespoon honey

Procedure:
1. Rinse the mixed berries and remove any stems.
2. Peel the lemon.
3. Add the mixed berries, peeled lemon, water, and honey to a blender.
4. Blend until well combined and smooth.

5. Pour the mixture into a glass and enjoy the detoxifying and tangy flavors of this berry detox drink.

35. **Apricot Energizer**:

Ingredients:
- 2 apricots
- 1 cup kale
- 1 green apple
- 1/2 lemon (peeled)

Procedure:
1. Wash the kale thoroughly.
2. Remove the pits from the apricots and cut them into smaller pieces.
3. Core the green apple and cut it into pieces.
4. Peel the lemon.
5. Juice the apricots, kale, green apple, and peeled lemon together.
6. Mix well and savor the energizing and vitamin-rich blend of this apricot elixir.

While aging is a natural process, antioxidants play a crucial role in combating oxidative stress and reducing cellular damage. By regularly consuming antioxidant-rich juices, you can provide your body with a concentrated dose of essential nutrients, promote skin health, support brain and heart health, and protect against age-related diseases.

CHAPTER FIVE

GAINING ENERGY THROUGH JUICING

The food we consume plays a crucial role in providing the energy needed for our daily activities. Our bodies require a balance of macronutrients, such as carbohydrates, proteins, and fats, as well as essential vitamins and minerals to fuel our cells and maintain optimal energy levels. When we provide our bodies with a nutrient-dense diet, we can experience higher energy levels, improved focus, and enhanced overall well-being.

On the other hand, consuming a diet high in processed foods, sugary snacks, and unhealthy fats can lead to energy crashes, fatigue, and a lack of vitality. These foods are often low in nutrients and can cause fluctuations in blood sugar levels, resulting in temporary energy spikes followed by crashes.

Energy-Boosting Ingredients for Juicing

Juicing provides an excellent way to boost your energy levels by delivering a concentrated dose of essential nutrients directly to your cells. Incorporating specific ingredients into your juices can further enhance their energy-boosting properties. Consider the following crucial ingredients:

1. Leafy Greens: Leafy greens such as spinach, kale, and Swiss chard are rich in chlorophyll, which helps increase oxygen levels in the blood and improve energy production. They are also packed with vitamins, minerals, and antioxidants that support overall health and vitality.

2. Citrus Fruits: Citrus fruits like oranges, lemons, and grapefruits are high in vitamin C and other antioxidants. These fruits help fight oxidative stress in the body, reduce inflammation, and provide a natural energy boost. Additionally, their refreshing flavors can uplift your mood and increase alertness.

3. Berries: Berries such as strawberries, blueberries, and raspberries are loaded with antioxidants and phytochemicals that help protect cells from damage caused by free radicals. They are also a good source of fiber, which helps stabilize blood sugar levels and prevent energy crashes.

4. Ginger: Ginger has long been used as a natural remedy for boosting energy and improving digestion. It has stimulating properties that can increase circulation and provide a natural energy

lift. Ginger also possesses anti-inflammatory and antioxidant effects, supporting overall well-being.

5. Turmeric: Turmeric contains curcumin, a compound known for its anti-inflammatory and antioxidant properties. It can help reduce fatigue and support healthy energy levels. Adding a pinch of black pepper to turmeric can enhance its absorption and effectiveness.

6. Pineapple: Pineapple is rich in enzymes, such as bromelain, which aids digestion and reduces inflammation. It also provides natural sugars and essential vitamins, including vitamin C and manganese, which are involved in energy production pathways.

7. Coconut Water: Coconut water is a natural source of electrolytes, including potassium, magnesium, and sodium. These electrolytes help maintain proper hydration and support energy production. Coconut water can be used as a base for your juices or added to enhance their hydrating properties.

8. Chia Seeds: Chia seeds are tiny powerhouses of nutrition. They are rich in omega-3 fatty acids, fiber, and protein, which can help stabilize blood sugar levels, promote satiety, and provide sustained energy throughout the day. When added to juices, chia seeds also add a pleasant texture.

9. Matcha Green Tea: Matcha green tea powder contains caffeine and L-theanine, an amino acid known for its calming effects. The combination of caffeine and L-theanine provides a sustained and focused energy boost without the jitters often associated with coffee. Adding matcha powder to your juices can provide a natural energy lift.

10. Maca Powder: Maca powder is derived from a root vegetable known for its adaptogenic properties. It can help balance hormones, reduce stress, and increase energy levels. Maca powder has a slightly nutty flavor and can be added to your juices for an energizing boost.

By incorporating these energy-boosting ingredients into your juicing routine, you can create delicious and nutritious blends that support your overall vitality and well-being. Experiment with different combinations and listen to your body to discover the recipes that work best for you. Remember to consume your juices as part of a balanced diet and maintain a healthy lifestyle to experience the full benefits of increased energy and improved overall health.

35 invigorating recipes for increased energy

Here's a comprehensive guide to the ingredients and procedures for invigorating recipes for increased energy:

1. Green Power Boost:

Ingredients:
- 2 cups spinach
- 1 cucumber
- 2 celery stalks
- 1 green apple
- 1 lemon (peeled)

Procedure:
a. Wash all the ingredients thoroughly.
  b. Cut the cucumber, celery stalks, green apple, and lemon into chunks.
  c. Place all the ingredients in a juicer and extract the juice.
  d. Stir the juice well and serve chilled.

2. Tropical Energy Blast:

Ingredients:
- 1 cup pineapple chunks
- 1 ripe banana
- 1 orange (peeled)
- 1-inch ginger root

Procedure:

a. Peel the orange and ginger root.

 b. Cut the pineapple, banana, orange, and ginger into chunks.

c. Combine all of the ingredients in a blender.

d. Blend until smooth and creamy.

e. Pour into a glass and enjoy.

3. **Berry Burst**:

Ingredients:
- 1 cup strawberries
- 1 cup blueberries
- 1 cup raspberries
- 1 cup coconut water

Procedure:

a. Rinse all the berries under running water.

 b. In a blender, combine the strawberries, blueberries, raspberries, and coconut water.

c. Blend until smooth and well combined.

d. Pour into a glass and enjoy.

4. **Citrus Zing**:

Ingredients:
- 2 oranges (peeled)
- 1 grapefruit (peeled)
- 1 lime (peeled)
- 1 tablespoon honey

Procedure:

a. Peel the oranges, grapefruit, and lime.

b. Cut them into chunks.

c. In a blender, combine the citrus chunks and honey.

d. Blend until smooth and refreshing.

e. Pour into a glass and serve chilled.

5. **Beet Energizer**:

Ingredients:
- 1 beetroot (peeled)
- 2 carrots
- 1 green apple
- 1-inch turmeric root

Procedure:

a. Wash and peel the beetroot and carrots.

b. Cut them into pieces.

c. Cut the green apple and turmeric root into chunks.

d. Place all the ingredients in a juicer and extract the juice.

e. Stir the juice well and serve chilled.

6. **Energizing Carrot Blend**:

Ingredients:
- 4 carrots
- 1 orange (peeled)
- 1-inch ginger root
- 1 tablespoon chia seeds

Procedure:

a. Wash and peel the carrots, orange, and ginger root.

b. Cut them into pieces.

c. In a blender, combine the carrots, orange, ginger root, and chia seeds.

d. Blend until smooth and well combined.

e. Pour into a glass and enjoy.

7. **Green Goddess**:

Ingredients:
- 2 cups kale
- 1 cucumber
- 1 green apple
- 1 lemon (peeled)
- 1 tablespoon spirulina powder

Procedure:

a. Wash the kale, cucumber, green apple, and lemon.

b. Cut them into pieces.

c. Feed all the ingredients into a juicer and extract the juice.

d. Stir in the spirulina powder until well combined.

e. Serve chilled.

8. **Pineapple Spinach Delight**:

Ingredients:
- 1 cup spinach

- 1 cup pineapple chunks
- 1 green apple
- 1/2 cup coconut water

Procedure:
a. Wash the spinach and pineapple chunks.
b. Cut the green apple into chunks.
   c. In a blender, combine the spinach, pineapple chunks, green apple, and coconut water.
d. Blend until smooth and creamy.
e. Pour into a glass and enjoy.

9. Mango Tango:

Ingredients:
- 2 ripe mangoes
- 1 orange (peeled)
- 1 lime (peeled)
- 1 tablespoon flaxseed oil

Procedure:
a. Peel the mangoes, orange, and lime.
b. Cut them into chunks.
   c. In a blender, combine the mangoes, orange, lime, and flaxseed oil.
d. Blend until smooth and well combined.
e. Pour into a glass and serve chilled.

10. Watermelon Refresher:

Ingredients:
- 2 cups watermelon chunks

- 1 cup cucumber
- 1/2 cup fresh mint leaves
- 1 tablespoon lime juice

Procedure:
a. Cut the watermelon into chunks.
b. Peel the cucumber and cut it into pieces.
 c. In a blender, combine the watermelon chunks, cucumber, fresh mint leaves, and lime juice.
d. Blend until smooth and refreshing.
e. Pour into a glass and serve chilled.

11. **Super Berry Blend**:

Ingredients:
- 1 cup strawberries
- 1 cup blackberries
- 1 cup raspberries
- 1 cup almond milk

Procedure:
a. Rinse all the berries under running water.
  b. In a blender, combine the strawberries, blackberries, raspberries, and almond milk.
c. Blend until smooth and well combined.
d. Pour into a glass and enjoy.

12. **Ginger Turmeric Boost**:

Ingredients:
- 1-inch ginger root
- 1-inch turmeric root

- 2 carrots
- 1 orange (peeled)

Procedure:
  a. Wash and peel the ginger root, turmeric root, and carrots.
  b. Cut them into pieces.
  c. Cut the orange into chunks.
  d. Place all the ingredients in a juicer and extract the juice.
  e. Stir the juice well and serve chilled.

13. **Citrus Spinach Twist**:

Ingredients:
- 2 cups spinach
- 2 oranges (peeled)
- 1 lemon (peeled)
- 1 tablespoon honey

Procedure:
  a. Wash the spinach, oranges, and lemon.
  b. Cut them into chunks.
  c. In a blender, combine the spinach, oranges, lemon, and honey.
  d. Blend until smooth and refreshing.
  e. Pour into a glass and serve chilled.

14. **Green Kiwi Refuel**:

Ingredients:
- 2 kiwis

- 1 green apple
- 1 cucumber
- 1 cup coconut water

Procedure:
a. Peel the kiwis and cut them into chunks.

b. Cut the green apple and cucumber into pieces.

c. In a blender, combine the kiwis, green apple, cucumber, and coconut water.

d. Blend until smooth and well combined.

e. Pour into a glass and enjoy.

15. **Pomegranate Power Punch**:

Ingredients:
- 1 cup pomegranate seeds
- 1 cup spinach
- 1 green apple
- 1-inch ginger root

Procedure:
a. Rinse the pomegranate seeds and spinach under running water.

b. Cut the green apple and ginger root into chunks.

c. In a blender, combine the pomegranate seeds, spinach, green apple, and ginger root.

d. Blend until smooth and vibrant.

e. Pour into a glass and enjoy.

16. **Energizing Kale Cooler**:

Ingredients:
- 2 cups kale
- 1 cucumber
- 1 green apple
- 1 lime (peeled)

Procedure:

   a. Wash the kale, cucumber, green apple, and lime.

   b. Cut them into pieces.

   c. Feed all the ingredients into a juicer and extract the juice.

   d. Stir the juice well and serve chilled.

17. **Tropical Green Burst**:

Ingredients:
- 1 cup pineapple chunks
- 1 cup mango chunks
- 2 cups spinach
- 1 cup coconut water

Procedure:

   a. Rinse the spinach under running water.

   b. Cut the pineapple and mango into chunks.

   c. In a blender, combine the pineapple chunks, mango chunks, spinach, and coconut water.

   d. Blend until smooth and creamy.

   e. Pour into a glass and enjoy.

18. Carrot Orange Splash:

Ingredients:
- 4 carrots
- 2 oranges (peeled)
- 1 lemon (peeled)
- 1 tablespoon hemp seeds

Procedure:
   a. Wash and peel the carrots, oranges, and lemon.
   b. Cut them into pieces.
   c. In a blender, combine the carrots, oranges, lemon, and hemp seeds.
   d. Blend until smooth and well combined.
   e. Pour into a glass and enjoy.

19. Berry Banana Blend:

Ingredients:
- 1 cup of mixed berries (strawberries, blueberries, and raspberries)
- 1 ripe banana
- 1 cup almond milk
- 1 tablespoon honey

Procedure:
   a. Rinse the mixed berries under running water.
   b. Peel the ripe banana.
   c. In a blender, combine the mixed berries, ripe banana, almond milk, and honey.
   d. Blend until smooth and creamy.

e. Pour into a glass and enjoy.

20. **Ginger Pear Revitalizer**:

Ingredients:
- 1 pear
- 1-inch ginger root
- 2 cups spinach
- 1 cup coconut water

Procedure:
   a. Rinse the pear and spinach under running water.
   b. Cut the pear and ginger root into chunks.
   c. In a blender, combine the pear, ginger root, spinach, and coconut water.
   d. Blend until smooth and well combined.
   e. Pour into a glass and serve chilled.

21. **Green Energy Refresher**:

Ingredients:
- 2 cups kale
- 1 cucumber
- 1 green apple
- 1 lemon (peeled)
- 1 tablespoon chia seeds

Procedure:
   a. Wash the kale, cucumber, green apple, and lemon.
   b. Cut them into pieces.

c. Feed all the ingredients into a juicer and extract the juice.

d. Stir in the chia seeds until well combined.

e. Serve chilled.

22. **Mango Spinach Surprise**:

Ingredients:
- 2 cups spinach
- 2 ripe mangoes
- 1 lime (peeled)
- 1 tablespoon flaxseed oil

Procedure:

a. Rinse the spinach under running water.

b. Peel the mangoes and cut them into chunks.

c. In a blender, combine the spinach, ripe mangoes, lime, and flaxseed oil.

d. Blend until smooth and vibrant.

e. Pour into a glass and enjoy.

23. **Zesty Carrot Ginger Boost**:

Ingredients:
- 4 carrots
- 1-inch ginger root
- 1 orange (peeled)
- 1 tablespoon honey

Procedure:

a. Wash and peel the carrots, ginger root, and orange.

b. Cut them into pieces.

c. In a blender, combine the carrots, ginger root, orange, and honey.

d. Blend until smooth and refreshing.

e. Pour into a glass and serve chilled.

24. **Blueberry Bliss**:

Ingredients:
- 2 cups blueberries
- 1 ripe banana
- 1 cup almond milk
- 1 tablespoon almond butter

Procedure:

a. Rinse the blueberries under running water.

b. Peel the ripe banana.

c. In a blender, combine the blueberries, ripe banana, almond milk, and almond butter.

d. Blend until smooth and creamy.

e. Pour into a glass and enjoy.

25. **Energizing Green Detox**:

Ingredients:
- 2 cups spinach
- 1 cucumber
- 2 celery stalks
- 1 green apple
- 1 lemon (peeled)

Procedure:

a. Wash the spinach, cucumber, celery stalks, green apple, and lemon.

b. Cut them into pieces.

c. Feed all the ingredients into a juicer and extract the juice.

d. Stir the juice well and serve chilled.

26. Pineapple Ginger Refuel:

Ingredients:
- 1 cup pineapple chunks
- 1-inch ginger root
- 2 cups spinach
- 1 cup coconut water

Procedure:

a. Rinse the spinach under running water.

b. Cut the pineapple and ginger root into chunks.

c. In a blender, combine the pineapple chunks, ginger root, spinach, and coconut water.

d. Blend until smooth and well combined.

e. Pour into a glass and enjoy.

27. Citrus Beet Blast:

Ingredients:
- 1 beetroot (peeled)
- 2 oranges (peeled)
- 1 grapefruit (peeled)
- 1 tablespoon chia seeds

Procedure:

a. Wash and peel the beetroot, oranges, and grapefruit.

b. Cut them into pieces.

c. In a blender, combine the beetroot, oranges, grapefruit, and chia seeds.

d. Blend until smooth and vibrant.

e. Pour into a glass and serve chilled.

28. Kale Mango Powerhouse:

Ingredients:
- 2 cups kale
- 2 ripe mangoes
- 1 lime (peeled)
- 1 tablespoon hemp seeds

Procedure:
a. Rinse the kale under running water

b. Peel the ripe mangoes and cut them into chunks.

c. In a blender, combine the kale, ripe mangoes, lime, and hemp seeds.

d. Blend until smooth and well combined.

e. Pour into a glass and enjoy.

29. Green Apple Elixir:

Ingredients:
- 2 green apples
- 1 cucumber
- 1 cup spinach

- 1-inch ginger root

Procedure:
    a. Wash the green apples, cucumber, spinach, and ginger root.
    b. Cut them into pieces.
    c. Feed all the ingredients into a juicer and extract the juice.
    d. Stir the juice well and serve chilled.

30. **Berry Beet Boost**:

Ingredients:
- 1 beetroot (peeled)
-1 cup of mixed berries (strawberries, blueberries, and raspberries)
- 1 orange (peeled)
- 1 tablespoon flaxseed oil

Procedure:
    a. Wash and peel the beetroot and orange.
    b. Rinse the mixed berries under running water.
    c. In a blender, combine the beetroot, mixed berries, orange, and flaxseed oil.
    d. Blend until smooth and vibrant.
    e. Pour into a glass and enjoy.

31. **Citrus Spinach Kick**:

Ingredients:
- 2 cups spinach
- 2 oranges (peeled)

- 1 lemon (peeled)
- 1 tablespoon honey

Procedure:
a. Wash the spinach, oranges, and lemon.
b. Cut them into chunks.
c. In a blender, combine the spinach, oranges, lemon, and honey.
d. Blend until smooth and refreshing.
e. Pour into a glass and serve chilled.

32. **Tropical Kale Twist**:

Ingredients:
- 2 cups kale
- 1 cup pineapple chunks
- 1 ripe banana
- 1 cup coconut water

Procedure:
a. Wash the kale and pineapple chunks.
b. Peel the ripe banana.
c. In a blender, combine the kale, pineapple chunks, ripe banana, and coconut water.
d. Blend until smooth and creamy.
e. Pour into a glass and enjoy.

33. **Carrot Turmeric Refresher**:

Ingredients:
- 4 carrots
- 1-inch turmeric root

- 1 orange (peeled)
- 1 tablespoon almond butter

Procedure:
  a. Wash and peel the carrots, turmeric root, and orange.
  b. Cut them into pieces.
  c. In a blender, combine the carrots, turmeric root, orange, and almond butter.
  d. Blend until smooth and refreshing.
  e. Pour into a glass and serve chilled.

34. **Watermelon Mint Energizer**:

Ingredients:
- 2 cups watermelon chunks
- 1 cup spinach
- 1/2 cup fresh mint leaves
- 1 tablespoon lime juice

Procedure:
  a. Cut the watermelon into chunks.
  b. Rinse the spinach under running water.
  c. In a blender, combine the watermelon chunks, spinach, fresh mint leaves, and lime juice.
  d. Blend until smooth and refreshing.
  e. Pour into a glass and serve chilled.

35. **Mango Coconut Zinger**:

Ingredients:
- 2 ripe mangoes

- 1 cup coconut water
- 1 lime (peeled)
- 1 tablespoon chia seeds

Procedure:
a. Peel the ripe mangoes and cut them into chunks.
b. In a blender, combine the ripe mangoes, coconut water, lime, and chia seeds.
c. Blend until smooth and well combined.
d. Pour into a glass and enjoy.

These invigorating recipes are packed with nutrients and are perfect for boosting your energy levels. For the greatest results, keep in mind to use high-quality, fresh ingredients. Enjoy these delicious and revitalizing drinks!

CHAPTER SIX

TIPS AND TRICKS FOR SUCCESSFUL JUICING

Juicing has grown in popularity as a method to include fruits and vegetables in a balanced diet. To make the most of your juicing experience, it's essential to follow some tips and tricks for successful juicing. This comprehensive guide will cover various aspects, including storing and preserving juices, making juicing a consistent part of your daily regimen, troubleshooting common juicing issues, and safety precautions and best practices.

1. Choose fresh and high-quality produce: Select ripe fruits and vegetables for juicing to ensure maximum flavor and nutrient content. Look for fresh, vibrant, and organic options whenever possible.

2. Wash your produce thoroughly: Before juicing, make sure to wash your fruits and vegetables properly to remove any dirt, pesticides, or contaminants. This step is essential for maintaining good hygiene and ensuring the safety of your juice.

3. Mix and match ingredients: Experiment with different combinations of fruits, vegetables, and

herbs to create unique flavors and maximize nutritional benefits. Mixing leafy greens with sweeter fruits can help balance the taste and increase nutrient density.

4. Prep your produce: Cut larger fruits and vegetables into smaller pieces to fit your juicer's feed chute easily. Removing any hard pits, seeds, or tough skins is also recommended for smoother juicing.

5. Alternate soft and hard ingredients: To optimize juicer performance, alternate between soft and hard produce while feeding them into the juicer. This technique helps prevent clogging and ensures efficient extraction.

6. Drink your juice immediately: Freshly made juice is the most nutritious and flavorful. Aim to consume your juice within 15-20 minutes of juicing to retain its maximum nutritional value. Exposure to air and light can cause oxidation, leading to nutrient loss.

7. Clean your juicer immediately: After each use, disassemble your juicer and clean all the parts thoroughly. Leaving the juicer uncleaned can lead to residue buildup and make subsequent cleaning more difficult.

8. Incorporate pulp into recipes: Don't discard the leftover pulp! It can be used in various recipes such

as soups, smoothies, muffins, or composted as a nutrient-rich addition to your garden.

9. Stay hydrated: While juicing is a great way to consume a variety of fruits and vegetables, it's important to remember that it's not a replacement for water. Drink plenty of water throughout the day to stay hydrated and support overall well-being.

Storing and Preserving Your Juices

1. Drink fresh juices whenever possible: Freshly made juice is the most nutritious and flavorful. However, if you need to store juice for later consumption, follow these guidelines.

2. Use airtight containers: Transfer your juice to airtight glass containers or bottles to minimize exposure to oxygen and preserve freshness.

3. Refrigerate promptly: Immediately refrigerate your juice after juicing to slow down the oxidation process and maintain the quality. Cold temperatures help slow down the growth of bacteria and enzymes that can spoil the juice.

4. Fill containers to the top: To minimize air contact and preserve the nutrients, fill the containers to the brim, leaving minimal headspace.

5. Consume within 24-48 hours: Freshly made juice should ideally be consumed within 24-48 hours for optimal taste and nutrition. The longer the juice sits, the more it may degrade in quality.

6. Freeze for longer storage: If you need to store juice for an extended period, freezing is an option. Pour the juice into ice cube trays or freezer-safe containers and freeze. Thaw the frozen juice in the refrigerator overnight before consuming.

Make Juicing a Consistent Part of Your Daily Regimen

1. Establish a routine: Set a specific time of the day for juicing to make it a regular habit. Whether it's in the morning, as a midday snack, or part of your evening routine, consistency is key.

2. Plan your ingredients: Stock up on a variety of fruits and vegetables so you always have options available for juicing. Create a shopping list and ensure your kitchen is well-stocked with fresh produce.

3. Prep in advance: Wash, cut, and portion your fruits and vegetables in advance, so they're ready to be juiced when needed. Prepping ahead of time saves time and makes juicing more convenient.

4. Set realistic goals: Determine your juicing goals and make them achievable. Start with smaller portions or incorporate one juice a day into your routine, then gradually increase as you feel comfortable.

5. Keep a juicing journal: Track your progress, including the recipes you enjoy, the effects you notice, and any changes in your overall well-being. This journal can help you stay motivated and identify what works best for you.

Troubleshooting Common Juicing Issues

1. Clogging: If your juicer gets clogged, it may be due to overloading or using fibrous ingredients. Cut produce into smaller pieces and alternate between soft and hard ingredients to prevent clogging.

2. Foam: Some juicers produce foam, which is a natural result of the juicing process. To reduce foam, skim it off the top of your juice before consuming or use a strainer to strain the juice after juicing.

3. Separation: Separation is common in freshly made juices. Simply give the juice a gentle stir before consuming to mix the layers back together.

4. Bitter taste: Certain ingredients, like citrus peels or bitter greens, can contribute to a bitter taste. Adjust the amount of these ingredients or balance them with sweeter fruits to achieve a more palatable flavor.

5. Pulp in juice: If you prefer pulp-free juice, strain it through a fine-mesh sieve or use a juicer with a built-in strainer. Alternatively, you can leave the pulp in for added fiber and nutrients.

Safety Precautions and Best Practices

1. Follow manufacturer instructions: Always read and follow the instructions provided by your juicer's manufacturer to ensure safe and proper usage.

2. Wash hands and equipment: Wash your hands thoroughly before handling produce and cleaning your juicer. Clean all juicing equipment, including cutting boards, knives, and juicer parts, after each use.

3. Use a stable surface: Place your juicer on a stable and flat surface to prevent accidents or damage. Ensure that the juicer is securely locked in place before operation.

4. Avoid overloading the juicer: Do not overload the juicer with excessive amounts of produce, as it can strain the motor and lead to malfunctions.

5. Unplug when not in use: After juicing, unplug the juicer from the power source and allow it to cool before disassembling for cleaning.

6. Store sharp blades safely: When handling and storing the blades or cutting components of your juicer, use caution to avoid accidental cuts. Store them in a secure place away from children's reach.

7. Listen to your body: If you have any underlying health conditions or concerns, consult with a healthcare professional or registered dietitian before making significant changes to your diet or juicing regimen.

By following these tips, storing your juices properly, making juicing a consistent part of your routine, troubleshooting common issues, and practicing safety precautions, you can enjoy the benefits of juicing in a safe and effective manner. Happy juicing!

CHAPTER SEVEN

FREQUENTLY ASKED QUESTIONS (FAQS); Answers to common questions about juicing

1. Is juicing better than eating whole fruits and vegetables?

While juicing extracts the liquid and nutrients from fruits and vegetables, it does remove the fiber content found in whole produce. Fiber is essential for digestion and maintaining a healthy gut. Both juicing and eating whole fruits and vegetables have their benefits. Juicing allows for quick nutrient absorption, while eating whole produce provides the added benefits of fiber and chewing, which aids in digestion. It's recommended to incorporate a balance of both juicing and consuming whole fruits and vegetables for a well-rounded diet.

2. Can I juice every day?

Yes, you can juice every day. However, it's essential to listen to your body and adjust your juicing routine to meet your individual needs. Juicing can be a healthy addition to your daily diet, but it should not replace whole foods entirely. It's best to consult with a healthcare professional or registered dietitian to ensure that juicing aligns with your specific dietary requirements.

3. Can juicing help with weight loss?

Juicing can support weight loss as part of a balanced diet and active lifestyle. It provides a concentrated source of nutrients with fewer calories, which can help control cravings and promote overall health. But it's crucial to keep in mind that juicing is not a miracle weight-loss cure-all. It should be combined with a well-rounded diet that includes a variety of whole foods and regular exercise.

4. Can juicing detoxify my body?

Juicing is often associated with detoxification, but it's important to understand that the body naturally detoxifies itself through the liver, kidneys, and other organs. Juicing can provide a boost of nutrients and hydration that supports the body's natural detoxification processes. However, be cautious of extreme or prolonged juice detoxes, as they may not provide adequate calories and nutrients for long-term health. It's advisable to focus on incorporating juicing as part of a balanced and sustainable lifestyle.

5. Can I store juice for later consumption?

Freshly made juice is recommended for optimal taste and nutrient content. However, if you need to store juice for later consumption, it's best to refrigerate it immediately in an airtight container to minimize oxidation and nutrient loss. Fresh juices can generally be stored in the refrigerator for up to 24-48 hours. If you require longer storage, freezing the juice in ice cube trays or freezer-safe containers is an option. Thaw the frozen juice in the refrigerator overnight before consuming.

6. Should I drink juice on an empty stomach?

There is no strict rule regarding when to consume juice. Some people prefer to drink it on an empty stomach in the morning to allow for quick nutrient absorption. Others may enjoy it as a snack or alongside a meal. Ultimately, it depends on personal preference and how your body responds. However, it's important to listen to your body and avoid consuming large amounts of juice in one sitting, as it can lead to spikes in blood sugar levels.

7. Can I juice if I have diabetes or other medical conditions?

If you have specific medical conditions, such as diabetes, it's important to consult with a healthcare professional or registered dietitian before making any significant changes to your diet, including juicing. They can provide personalized guidance and recommendations based on your individual needs, helping you create a juicing plan that aligns with your health goals and medical conditions.

8. Can children and pregnant women consume fresh juice?

Fresh juice can be enjoyed by children and pregnant women, but it's essential to exercise caution and moderation. For children, it's important to introduce juices gradually and ensure they are consuming a well-rounded diet that includes whole fruits and vegetables. Pregnant women should consult with their healthcare provider regarding specific dietary guidelines and any restrictions. It's generally recommended to prioritize whole fruits and vegetables over excessive juice consumption during pregnancy.

9. Can I juice herbs and spices?

Yes, herbs and spices can be added to juices to enhance flavors and provide additional health benefits. Common herbs and spices used in juicing include ginger, turmeric, mint, basil, and parsley.

However, use them in moderation and be mindful of their potent flavors. Some herbs and spices may have specific interactions with medications, so if you are on medication, it's advisable to consult with a healthcare professional or registered dietitian before incorporating them into your juices.

10. Can I use a blender instead of a juicer?

Blenders can be used to make blended smoothies that retain the fiber content of fruits and vegetables. While blenders can create thick and nutritious beverages, they don't separate the juice from the pulp like a juicer does. If you prefer a smoother juice-like consistency, a juicer is recommended. However, blending can be a suitable alternative if you prefer to consume whole fruits and vegetables.

It's important to note that these answers provide general information, and individual circumstances may vary. For personalized advice and guidance, it's always best to consult with a healthcare professional or registered dietitian who can consider your specific needs, goals, and medical history.

CHAPTER EIGHT

CONCLUSION

Embracing the power of juicing for a healthier and more vibrant life the essential guide to juicing for beginners has provided a comprehensive and invaluable resource for individuals looking to incorporate juicing into their lives. With over 100 juicing recipes for weight loss, detoxification, preventing aging, and gaining energy, this guide offers a wide array of options to suit various health goals and taste preferences.

Juicing has been shown to have numerous benefits, including weight loss, detoxification, increased energy levels, and slowing down the aging process. By harnessing the power of fruits, vegetables, herbs, and spices, juicing allows you to extract the vital nutrients, vitamins, minerals, and antioxidants present in these natural ingredients.

This guide offers a diverse range of recipes, allowing beginners to experiment and discover the flavors and health benefits that resonate with them. Whether you're seeking weight loss, detoxification, an energy boost, or to promote youthful skin, the recipes provided cover a wide spectrum of needs and tastes.

For weight loss, the guide highlights key ingredients such as leafy greens, citrus fruits, and metabolism-boosting spices. These ingredients not only aid in weight management but also provide essential nutrients to support overall health and well-being.

To promote detoxification, the guide emphasizes the inclusion of ingredients like beets, lemon, and greens that are known for their detoxifying properties. These recipes can help eliminate toxins from the body and support the natural detoxification processes.

This guide also recognizes the desire to slow down the aging process and maintain youthful vitality. Recipes rich in antioxidants, such as berries, green tea, and cruciferous vegetables, can help combat oxidative stress and reduce the signs of aging.

In addition to the extensive recipe collection, this guide provides valuable information on the role of juicing in weight management, detoxification, and energy enhancement. It offers practical tips and techniques for successful juicing, including ingredient selection, preparation, and storage. By addressing common concerns and providing safety precautions, the guide ensures that beginners can embark on their juicing journey with confidence and knowledge.

In conclusion, the essential guide to juicing for beginners is a comprehensive and valuable resource for those seeking to harness the power of juicing for weight loss, detoxification, preventing aging, and gaining energy. With a wide variety of recipes, practical tips, and important information, this guide equips beginners with the tools they need to embark on a healthy and vibrant juicing lifestyle. By incorporating these recipes and practices into their daily routine, individuals can experience the transformative benefits of juicing and improve their overall health and well-being. Cheers to a vibrant and nourished life through the world of juicing!

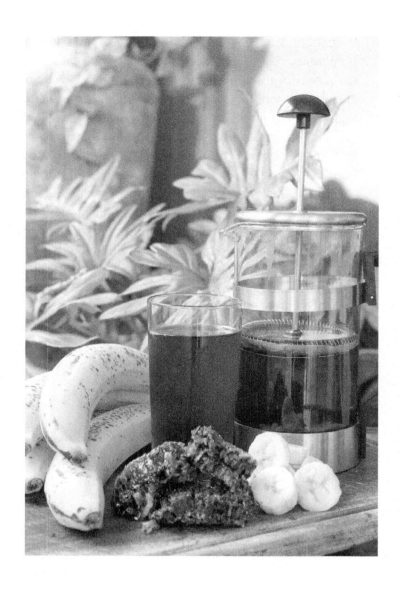

Printed in Great Britain
by Amazon

28717836R00076